Soon To Be DAD

Handbook For Expectant Fathers

By

P. A. Simon

Disclaimer

All the material contained in this book is provided for educational and informational purposes only. No responsibility can be taken for any results or outcomes resulting from the use of this material.

While every attempt has been made to provide information that is both accurate and effective, the author does not assume any responsibility for the accuracy or use/misuse of this information.

Second edition: May 2020

ISBN: 9798645554279

Contents

To my wife for her strength and perseverance.

To my beloved son for the joy and motivation, he gives.

INTRODUCTION

I have a son! What a joy! I've always wanted to be a responsible parent, which is why I've decided that I need to prepare for being a dad the best possible. If you reached for this book, I'm sure you're planning on becoming a father or soon will be one. I remember that feeling really well. The excitement with a pinch of terror. You need to remember that waiting for a child and fatherhood is not a terrible thing; however, it is vital to prepare well. This guidebook will undoubtedly help you do that. Many pregnancy books are available on the market, but for the most part, they are meant for women. There is nothing peculiar about it, in all ends, it's women who get pregnant. So why did I decide to write a guidebook on pregnancy and fatherhood? The answer is simple.

On the one hand, I felt an emotional need to describe this wonderful time in my life. On the other hand, I wanted to share my knowledge and experience so that the reader, as a future parent, does not have to search for relevant information in multi-page books. Times are changing, and conscious and responsible men would also like to prepare for these beautiful nine months and the birth of a child. They just want to participate, often with the same or sometimes more significant commitment than future moms.

This guide is therefore written for future dads, but it can undoubtedly also be recommended to future moms, too. Why is that? Not only to find out what concerns lie in the head of a partner or husband but above all, because it is a collection of selected, that is, the most critical information (from the male point of view), which both future parents should know about.

You must have a lot of questions on your mind. Are you wondering if you'll be a good father? How can you support your partner? What tests should be performed during pregnancy, and should you participate? How to start preparing for the birth of a child? What should you pay attention to when buying a baby stroller? Which crib to purchase and which mattress will be the best? How to prepare for the emotional fluctuations of a partner during pregnancy? Is there anything you don't know that needs to be dealt with? There are a lot of questions and doubts I will try to dispel in this book. You've already taken the first step since you're looking for information on parenting prep. This means you are a responsible person and want to provide the best care of your wife and child. I'm the same. I looked for information wherever I could, including the Internet, although I do not think forums always work. I have read several few hundred-page books written by eminent authorities in the fields gynecology and obstetrics, met with gynecologists and obstetricians, consulted necessary products for infants with retailers, representatives of companies and even certification bodies, read the results of the latest research, participated in the birth school and 'Safe toddler' workshop.[1]

I filtered out all this knowledge, excluding insignificant information, combined it with my own experience, and described it in this guidebook, which is meant to be a guide and source of selected data for you, as a future well-informed dad. This book can also be a great motivator for making changes in your life. Exactly, there is no better motivator than your own child, and I describe it based on my story.

In the book, I'm going to tell you my story so you can find out what kind of situation I was in. Yours might be similar. You can also find very personal confessions about the pregnancy problems my wife and I experienced. I try to support cold facts with my own experience, and when describing strategic accessories for your child, I rely on the consultations I have conducted and indicate what you should pay attention to. They were not hasty decisions. I based them on personal thoughts and analyses.

Enjoy reading!

---

[1] 'Safe toddler' is a series of workshops for pregnant women, which take place in my country (topics include first aid in emergencies in infants, safety of toddlers on the move, safety and first aid to pregnant women).

MY STORY

Twenty years earlier

I met my wife 20 years ago. I was 16 at the time. My parents and I moved from the country to a nearby town. This was in May, which is why I spent the entire last month of my primary school commuting to the countryside. Moving house could not have happened at a better time for me. Graduating from elementary school was inevitably connected with starting secondary school in the same town. Therefore I did not have to say goodbye to my friends and meet new people during elementary school. I spent the first holiday in a new place with my old friends. My grandmother has always lived in the country, so I had a place to stay. In September, I started studying in junior high school and started getting to know people from my area. Back in the summer, I was introduced to the neighbors in my part of the apartment building. They turned out to be social enough to invite my sister and me to play together. I was a bit intimidated. I am an open person, not ashamed to meet people, but the new environment blocked me, and I felt uncomfortable. Over time, as I met more and more people, I had more opportunities to hang out together and kill time. I met my wife, Anna, at my neighbor's. Of course, at the time, I had no idea that we would share something in the future. It wasn't until after a few years of the relationship when she told me she was competing with my neighbor for me. But before we became a couple, we spent time among mutual friends. What I particularly remember was our New Year's Eve at my friend's in the country. After all these years, I am not even able to indicate a specific date from which Anna and I were no longer just friends, and our relationship has turned into a crush and a bond. I'm deliberately writing about infatuation because love, as such, came much later. To my horror, we even had a break-up year, but today I may say this proves we have always meant to be together.

We just had to grow up to understand the situation. I smile at myself when I think about our thoughts and our approach to living together, marriage, and children. I correctly remember Anne saying she could not imagine herself in a wedding dress. We had a similar approach to children. We were just too young at the time and had different priorities. The most important thing for us was education and getting a job. Marriage and children were somewhere at the end of our plan. A plan we have not come to yet. It was high school time. We were both thinking about college. Anne is two years younger than me, so I was the one who paved the way. I started my first studies at German philology. The choice was simple – I got the best results in German at school, and this was a clear educational choice. Of course, I did not imagine myself being a teacher, but luckily I live in an extraordinarily touristic and not very industrialized region. The region has always been visited by a lot of tourists, mostly from Germany. I thought working in the HoReCa industry[2] would be the right choice. To this day, I believe that German studies were the right choice. My knowledge of foreign languages made it much easier for me to get a casual job as a waiter or bartender in nearby hotels where many tourists stayed during my studies. I am quite sure, my ability to communicate in foreign languages was my main asset. It was just the reason I could start my first full-time job at a production company where I was involved in international trade.

We did not have an easy life, but we did not like to complain about it, either. Admittedly, my parents paid for my full-time studies (a private university), but they also sacrificed a lot to afford it. Mostly my mom, who, for as long as I can remember, did a lot of overtime work at two different companies and also often took the work home. She was an accountant, and luckily the number of people interested in her services was quite significant. I did not want to burden my parents financially. Aiming at earning for my needs, at the age of sixteen, I started taking holiday jobs. Thus, for three consecutive years, I spent my vacation working for a beverage and alcohol wholesaler. At the age of nineteen, after getting to college, I took up a job as a waiter at a holiday resort located about 6 or 7 miles from my town. This experience enabled me to get another job as a waiter at a hotel with a much better reputation. I started full-time studies. I commuted to college 26 miles by train every day, came back in the afternoon, and worked as a waiter from 5 p.m. to 11 p.m. The next morning I went to college, then I came back to the hotel, and this continued for a few

---

[2] HoReCa is a popular term for the hotel and catering sector. The acronym comes from the words: **Ho**tel, **Re**staurant, **Ca**tering.

years. This sequence of events taught me humility and respect for the money I earned.

After graduation, I changed my employer and started working full-time at a four-star hotel. I remember perfectly well that on the first day, after talking to other waiters, I learned about the standard rate at which new employees work. On the second day, I went to the hotel owners, to whom I presented my previous experience in the industry, informed them about my knowledge of foreign languages, and my proposal for a minimum rate at which I can work with them. It was 60% higher than the generally accepted standard for new employees. I have never had a problem communicating with others or with proper arguments; therefore, I suppose my proposal was accepted. However, I did not tell my colleagues that I had managed to negotiate a better remuneration.

My wife got a harder kick from life, though. Her parents couldn't afford to pay for college, especially since her father died in the early years of our relationship. Her mother worked to support the house and two sons. I deliberately did not mention Ann here because after graduating from secondary school, she found a job at a local shop. This way, she could earn money for further education and her needs. She first enrolled in a cosmetology course. However, she felt it was inadequate and wanted to study at a university. It was her idea to start studies together at the same school. She studied in the field of rehabilitation pedagogy, and I decided to follow the general pedagogy program. We completed three-year bachelor studies together and enrolled in two-year master studies. For five years, we followed the extramural plan at weekends, so we could work on weekdays. During our studies, we managed to obtain a scholarship for excellent academic results five times in a row, so it was an additional influx of cash for us.

In 2008, my parents got divorced, and this uncomfortable situation motivated me to buy an apartment and move out of the house. I took out a mortgage and moved in with my wife. This was a time when we were still studying, so official marriage or a child was not a priority for us. At some point, I felt the need to formalize the relationship, which is why in the second year of our mutual life, I decided to propose. There's a funny story involved because I wanted the engagement to be very original. I bought a ring and packed it in five or six boxes. The smaller box was wrapped in a bigger one, and so on. I eventually ended up with a huge box. I asked a friend, who worked as a courier, to deliver a package to my future wife, pretending, of course, that we had not known each other. I marked Ann's aunt from across the country as the sender of the package. When the courier called the intercom, I thought my heart would pop out of my chest. Ann asked me to pick up a package. I asked the courier how come they were still working this late. Ann did not even suspect we had known each other. I picked up a package. She glanced at the sender, and she was pleased to find out that her aunt had sent her something. She began to open box after box, laughing and wondering who could pack it this way. Eventually, in the smallest box, she found a ring in a jewelry gift box. She opened the box and said: *Oh, this is the ring auntie and I talked about the last time we met. It belonged to her great-grandmother and was passed down from generation to generation.* I laughed and told her it was my ring and asked her to give it back. She insisted it was the ring from the auntie, so under high stress and excitement, I took the ring, knelt down, and proposed. Until now, when I think about it, I laugh under my breath.

Of course, none of our parents offered to finance or contribute to the cost of our wedding and wedding reception (even if they did, we would not accept it), and we thought taking out a loan to host a one-day reception was a bad idea. So we decided to tighten our belts and save for this great day, which finally came on September 2, 2016. We organized the whole reception ourselves, very meticulously, but I will not go into details. The plan was fully implemented. We graduated from university, found jobs we were happy with, so it was time to have a baby.

Two years before pregnancy

Getting pregnant is no easy for everyone

A child is a great gift, but not meant for everyone. Few people understand those who have problems getting pregnant or for medical reasons cannot have children at all. Not being able to get pregnant is a terrible feeling, and I do not wish it on anyone. It is only when the problem affects our loved ones or us that we begin to realize what helplessness is. The growing desire to have a child is not helpful, either. I remember meeting a man about my age in a hospital elevator. We were both on our way to the cafe, and our conversation went on for about half an hour.

The topic quickly escalated to problems with getting pregnant. The man told me his story, which included almost a five-year battle for pregnancy, which ended in the birth of a baby. Conception was possible only through in vitro fertilization. They finally succeeded on the sixth try. Of course, it took months in the endless trials, doctor's appointments, and tests for it to happen. I will remember his story for the rest of my life. The longing for a child and all the problems they encountered along the way. We complained in agreement about the lack of government support in our country for people with similar issues. If you want to fight for the baby and need to use procedures such as in vitro, you have to be able to afford it. The cost they incurred was the equivalent of a new, middle-class car, but neither he nor I had any doubts as to whether it was worth it. What about the people who cannot afford it and want a baby more than anything else in their lives? I do not even want to think about it. The man I met is not planning on having more children, but he is thinking of couples in which one partner (or both, which is rare but possible) cannot have children for medical reasons. He and his wife decided to waive their right to frozen, remaining eggs for someone else to use. That way, they might make someone happy.

We knew we wanted to have a baby even before we got married. Of course, we were aware that we would not be young parents, which was quite typical 15–20 years ago. The average age of a pregnant woman at that time was 25, today it is 30. As I described above, we had other priorities, namely studies and work. In 2018, we began our efforts. As conscious prospective parents, we did a complete set of tests. My wife's tests were paramount because she has hypothyroidism and some non-surgical pituitary changes. We knew that both the thyroid gland and the pituitary gland are responsible for the production and secretion of hormones into the body, and hormonal disorders are critical in trying to get pregnant, as well as maintaining it. An abnormal hormone level may prevent pregnancy or cause miscarriage. We did tests of prolactin and TSH, hormones produced by the pituitary gland (TSH stimulates the thyroid gland to produce more hormones: T3 and T4). Their levels were regulated by medication. These are prescription drugs, so my wife was under constant care of both a gynecologist and an endocrinologist. Improper levels of lactogenic hormone or TSH can cause fetal defects, which is why it was so essential for us to normalize these levels. Of course, any future mother should see a gynecologist before the planned pregnancy. Your doctor will do an interview and arrange for the necessary tests to inform you of any contraindications. If the morphology results are not typical, the doctor will prescribe appropriate medication or recommend supplementation. In our case, in addition to thyroid problems, we were aware of issues with the secretion of prolactin, a hormone produced by the pituitary gland. Proper diet and supplementation are also of paramount importance. I will follow this topic in the next chapter.

My wife's vitals were normal, so were mine. However, despite our best efforts, we were unable to conceive. As the months went by, we became more and more irritated. There's not much in life that comes easy, but we were hoping the pregnancy wouldn't be a problem. Sometimes I joke that my wife is like a witch. Her hunches work in a lot of cases. Before we started our efforts, she said she felt we could do it at once. Unfortunately, that was not the case.

Our efforts

Six months have passed on trying to get pregnant. We couldn't understand why it didn't work out and why it affected us. There are so many unwanted babies born. Of course, even if unplanned, children are loved by their parents. I mean the unwanted ones that are given away, and yet – horror of horrors - killed. Why is it that in pathological families, a child is born after a child, and we cannot experience that happiness? We could not figure it out.

The gynecologist who had been taking care of Anne so far had no idea what might be causing it, so we decided to seek help on our own. The first thing we thought about was changing doctors. Just because one cannot help, it does not mean another cannot, either. We began our search. Considering specialists from all over the country, we focused on those nearby, so we did not have to go too far if it was not necessary. We found a doctor in the provincial city, 27 miles away from our place, who enjoyed great recognition among patients. He works as a deputy chief in the local hospital in the gynecologic and obstetrics ward. He also runs a private medical practice and co-owns a clinic that deals with infertility and problems with pregnancy. We thought he was the man. At the first visit, he did an interview, checked already available results of the tests, and examined my wife. He found no contraindications to pregnancy, but he was also unable to find the cause of the problem.

The first stage in fighting the problems with conception is the so-called monitoring, i.e., observing ovulation by vaginal ultrasound, on which I will elaborate more in the following chapters. This involves several doctor's visits, usually day after day, to see if eggs form and then whether their sheath (called Graafian follicle) bursts and releases the egg cell. The size of the eggs, read diameter, is also checked to see if it corresponds with a particular day of ovulation. In our case, there was usually one egg. Admittedly, sometimes its size was too small, sometimes too large, but it was always within limits. I remember the doctor saying on the right day of ovulation: today and tomorrow, try harder. And we were trying, but it did not work. In fact, the doctor did not even have to tell us when there was ovulation. We also knew when the bubble burst. Not all women do, but my wife knows and feels her body very well. She could sense ovulation, i.e., using the symptoms such as swollen breasts or the amount of mucus, and the rupture of the bubble itself, which is manifested by slight pain.

After five monitoring sessions, i.e., full menstrual cycles, due to suspicion of poor quality Graaf follicles, we moved to the next stage, i.e., pharmacological stimulation of ovulation. This step aims at stimulating ovaries to conduct the proper maturation of egg cells. Making it simple, this is the way to improve the quality of the egg cells.

The next stage, we were slowly preparing for, was checking the tubal patency of the fallopian tubes. This is a painful procedure for a woman, but it answers whether an egg cell released from the egg moves into the fallopian tube after the rupture of the Graafian follicle. The following stages include intrauterine insemination, i.e., administering the sperm of the partner directly into the womb of the woman and in vitro, i.e., extra-corporeal fertilization, in other words, combining ova with male reproductive cells in laboratory conditions and placing the embryo in the womb.

After the monitoring process started, I decided to test my semen. I did it without any persuasion from my wife. If you have problems similar to those described here, do not hesitate for a moment. I do not understand people who still stick to the historical theory today, which claims if there is a problem with getting pregnant, it is the woman's fault. If that is what you think, then you are wrong. In my case, the results of the semen test confirmed that all parameters assessing the sperm were correct. The high concentration of sperm in one milliliter of semen with a significant volume of ejaculate resulted in a very high number of available sperm in the entire volume of semen. The sperm were viable, moved correctly, and the absolute amount of sperm of the correct build was high. The excellent image was obscured by leukocytes, which in total significantly exceeded the permissible amount in one milliliter of semen. These symptoms may have suggested inflammation, which I was trying to eliminate.

And it worked

On-demand sex is not as pleasant as a spontaneous one. I guess I do not have to prove it. Unfortunately, we had to get used to it. Frustration was already at a very high level, so there were even arguments. The constant stress associated with our helplessness increased prolactin, a hormone that we regulated pharmacologically. Regardless of our well-being or possible quarrels, attempts at conception had to be made. Our close-ups have become mechanical. Sometimes we used to laugh about it. We had to do it, that's it. We bought pregnancy tests in bulk. Ovulation tests (yes, such tests are also available) were not necessary because – as I have already mentioned – my wife could feel her body perfectly. The monitoring carried out during each cycle, correctly informed us when ovulation occurred. This mechanical approach to sex was really irritating for us, it caused anxiety and stress, so we were in a kind of vicious circle.

Every month, we waited for the menstruation, and more specifically, we hoped it would not happen. I carefully observed my wife, hoping to see any signs of malaise that might indicate pregnancy. I remember that before I saw a positive pregnancy test, my wife had not felt like eating bread for a few days. Whether she was to eat a bun or some bakery products, she did not feel like eating it. I would be lying if I said that I did not hope this lack of appetite was due to pregnancy, but it was not accompanied by any nausea or reluctance to eat at all, so I was not entirely convinced. About 2-3 days before the pregnancy test, my wife was very sleepy. She would come home from work and get a nap for 30-60 minutes, which she had not done before. Now I am confident that the only symptoms of my wife's pregnancy were reluctance to eat pastry and weakness in the body manifested by the need for a nap during the day. You may find similar traits in your partner, but keep in mind that this is a very individual, and each woman shows different symptoms of pregnancy.

Anne started work before me, so it was natural for her to get out of bed earlier than me. One morning she ran into the bedroom with a test in her hand and said to me in a low but very excited voice: *Have a look cause I cannot see it right. Is the second line starting to appear here? It is hard to see, but it starts to show, doesn't it?* I was asleep, but I quickly got up, and I saw and confirmed that the second line was kind of foggy, but visible. We fell into each other's arms engulfed in such positive excitement that it is hard to describe in words. After all, after months of trying, we were finally pregnant.

UNDERSTAND PREGNANCY

You probably think you do not need any pregnancy theory at all, and it is only women who need it. This is not true. Especially if you want to understand a pregnant woman well and prepare for these nine months of waiting for a baby. Start by deepening your knowledge of pregnancy. Undoubtedly, it will ease meaningful conversations with the specialists you are going to meet now. If you decide to support your partner and accompany her during this nine-month journey, it is inevitable. Besides, impressing your friends with your knowledge of pregnancy is invaluable. So here it is.

Ovulation and insemination

I think all men are aware that women go through menstrual cycles. And I am sure they already know about the regular period that every woman goes through in her own way. Some of the women do not feel any discomfort, others are irritable, and some others feel great pain. For my wife, the pregnancy and months after giving birth, i.e., the period without menstruation, were kind to her in this respect.

At the end of menstruation, the follicle begins to develop. Its development is possible thanks to follicle-stimulating hormone, which also affects the ovaries placed at the end of the fallopian tubes. If it is beyond your imagination, take a look at the picture of the female reproductive system. Each ovary (there are two) usually releases one egg. Ovulation takes place alternately, i.e., one egg is released from one ovary and the next egg from the other. Approximately 20 eggs mature each month, but only one survives, the others wither. The level of estrogen, a hormone that affects, among other things, breast tissue, increases. Therefore, you may notice that your partner's breasts are much more sensitive before her menstrual period.

The info on the follicle state reaches the hypothalamus in the brain, and it is routed to the pituitary gland. The gland secretes the luteinizing hormone, which leads to the release of an egg about a day later. The egg pulls away from the bubble, and then ovulation begins. This usually happens on the 14th day of the cycle (the cycle counts from the first day of menstruation). Ovulation may occur a few days later or earlier. It is not a symptom of any disorder. In my wife's case, ovulation took place on days 10 or 11 of the cycle. When progesterone and estrogen levels fall below levels that allow the uterus to remain ready for embryonic attachment, the mucous membrane of the uterus begins to peel, causing bleeding. That is what menstruation is.

After reading the above paragraph, you probably think that our role as the core participants in the entire fertilization process is much simpler. But it only seems so. You should know that the likelihood of your sperm reaching the egg cell is very low. There are between 100 and 300 million sperm in the standard amount of semen secreted. Only about 200 reach the fallopian tubes, and only one will be able to fertilize an egg. During orgasm and ejaculation, the sperm enter the vagina, but the environment is not favorable because vaginal secretions have an acidic reaction. After about 5-10 minutes, the sperm reach the uterus and then the fallopian tubes, where they become very active. Once the sperm cell reaches the egg cell, it releases an acrosome from its head, which allows it to penetrate the egg cell. Other sperm cells also reach the egg cell, but the process of penetration takes about 24 hours, and only one can reach the oocyte (the deepest layer of the egg cell) where fertilization occurs.

Your role in conceiving a child

Already in the previous section, I explained to you that a man's participation in conceiving a child is not as simple as it seems at first glance. Remember, your fertility must be at a high level. Statistically, 1 in 10 men has various fertility issues. If you are planning on having a baby, I recommend making a full blood count. However, if your partner is having trouble getting pregnant for reasons not yet known to you, do not wait, just test the semen. Male infertility is referred to when fertilization does not occur during regular coitus without contraception. But do not worry too much, you can already improve your sperm quality by modifying your lifestyle, including your diet.

What should you focus on? Firstly: **physical activity.** You cannot avoid it. According to the World Health Organization, the minimum adult exercise dose should be 30 minutes of moderate exercise 5 times a week or 20 minutes of intensive training 3 times a week. At the same time, the WHO recommends minimizing sitting time to a maximum of two hours per day. It's best to keep your BMI[3] at 20-25 levels. Both too thin and too obese men may have semen of inferior quality.

Secondly: **proper diet**. It is best to use a balanced diet arranged by a specialist individually for a particular person. This is not necessary as long as you are aware of what healthy eating habits are. You can enrich your menu with a few products and eliminate or minimize unhealthy food. Unhealthy, i.e., processed food. Start reading the labels of the products you buy. If not all the label data is clear to you, I recommend using the facilities of today's world. I use an app, which, after scanning the barcode, shows the composition of a given product and informs which ingredients are healthy and recommended and which are not. I recommend limiting or giving up ready-made products, fast-foods, and snacks. Just do not get paranoid, it really will not hurt if you eat something unhealthy from time to time. I still stick to the rule that if I want to eat fast food, it is once a week (usually at the weekend).

---

[3] BMI - body mass index calculated by dividing body weight (kg) by the square of body height (m).

Male fertility is greatly influenced by zinc, which is associated with testosterone production. You can increase its amount in the body by eating, among others, red meat, fish, legumes, or pumpkin seeds. Vitamin E found in eggs and hazelnuts, and vitamin C found in citrus have a similar effect. Another ingredient that supports sperm production is selenium, and its excellent sources are brown rice, oats, pumpkin seeds, garlic, wheat, as well as milk, lean meat, and fish. I additionally introduced Brazil nuts to our diet, which improve fertility because they are an excellent source of selenium, calcium, magnesium, vitamin E, folic acid, and potassium. Just a few nuts a day should do. I also ate fresh vegetables with each meal because they are a source of antioxidants.

Thirdly: **quit smoking and reduce alcohol consumption**. You know very well that smoking is bad for you. It affects fertility and, like alcohol, reduces sperm motility as well as count.

Fourthly: **supplementation**. If you are unable to provide your body with a sufficient dose of the above-mentioned essential elements, you can use supplementation. It is best to consult a doctor or nutritionist about the appropriate supplements.

Pregnancy confirmation

The urine test is the most popular and the simplest and quickest way to confirm pregnancy. You can easily buy the test in pharmacies, drugstores, or other outlets. The urine test checks the level of hCG, an embryo (and later placenta) secreted hormone. You should know that urine tests can be considered reliable, but remember that the hCG level increases approximately seven days after fertilization, so wait patiently and perform the analysis within 8-10 days of the suspected date of conception. I have already written about the fact that our test showed a blurry second line, which is why my wife checked the blood at the lab to determine the level of hCG on the same day - this is the second method that can somehow confirm the result of the urine test. Blood hCG levels show norms and hCG values for women at different stages of the menstrual cycle, as well as standards for pregnant women, which determine hCG levels in a specific week of pregnancy. It is recommended (and we did so) to repeat the hCG blood test after a few days. Concentrations of this hormone increase at a tremendous rate in the first days and weeks of pregnancy, so a much higher value in the second test should give 100% certainty.

Proper diet and supplementation for women before and during pregnancy

If you are going to start eating healthily or have already introduced the appropriate eating habits described in the section *Your role in conceiving a child,* you should also encourage your partner to do so. She should focus on a healthy diet and the necessary supplementation at least three months before she plans to become pregnant. Once she is pregnant, her diet should be even more restrictive than yours. I'll get to the details in a moment.

From the moment of conception, everything the future mother eats will be broken down into tiny particles and enter the baby's bloodstream through the placenta. Please note that you do not need to deliver more than about 2,000-kilocalories per day in the first trimester. Anything that is eaten in excess will not be suitable for the developing baby and will simply be put aside as additional fat tissue. Women increase their weight by an average of about 30 pounds during nine months of pregnancy, but this is not the rule, so do not worry if weight gain is less or more significant. My wife gained 20 pounds. Of course, it had a lot to do with premature labor. If our son had been more patient and had not rushed into the world four weeks ahead of schedule, his weight would undoubtedly have increased. Different values of weight gain of pregnant women are given, however, averaging this data allows us to assume that the pregnancy is an additional weight of 24-35 pounds, which includes on average: the child (6-9 pounds), placenta (1.5 pounds), amniotic fluids (2 pounds), increased amount of maternal blood (3.3-4 pounds), fatty tissue of the mother (5.5-6.6 pounds), breasts of the mother (1-2 pounds), enlarged uterus (2 pounds), tissue fluids in the mother's body (4-5.5 pounds).

A common-sense approach should apply to the nutrition of a pregnant woman. Of course, you can try to stick to a strict diet, but life will quickly verify that. In many cases, the first trimester (the first three months of pregnancy) includes nausea and vomiting, so it is no surprise that in such a condition, it is not possible to maintain the previously set nutritional guidelines. As I said before, every pregnancy is different. In my wife's case, the first few days we did not know she was pregnant, she could not eat bread, but I do not recall her having any cravings that differed from the standard menu throughout her pregnancy. I am referring here to the urban legends of desires such as pickled cucumber with mayonnaise, or other non-standard combinations that a pregnant woman might want to have.

For a balanced diet, the right amount and source of protein, carbohydrates, and fats are essential. From the very beginning of pregnancy, the demand for protein, which is a necessary building block of muscles, bones, and connective tissues, increases by about 15-20% on average. Meat, poultry, fish, eggs, and dairy products should, therefore, constitute an indispensable part of the diet. When it comes to carbohydrates, we should divide them into simple and complex ones. Simple carbohydrates present low nutritional value, rapidly absorb into the bloodstream, giving an injection of energy, and quickly burn. Only fructose is an exception to this rule, and therefore pregnant women are advised to consume 4-5 portions of the fruit that also contain a large number of vitamins and a substantial amount of fiber. Complex carbohydrates are the basis for a well-balanced diet, as they take much longer to decompose than simple ones. In other words, energy is released more slowly, and the body needs to work more to burn them properly. Rice and pasta are good sources of complex carbohydrates, preferably wholegrain ones. Fats, on the other hand, provide the body with the necessary vitamins and participate in the construction of cell walls. They are divided into less healthy, so-called saturated, of animal origin and healthier, so-called unsaturated, which we can find in the fish and vegetables.

Minerals, mainly iron, calcium, and zinc, should be controlled too. Iron plays an essential role in our body because it is a component of hemoglobin that transports blood. During pregnancy, the amount of blood of a woman doubles, and the needs of the child also matter here. It is, therefore, not surprising that you need to increase your iron intake to avoid anemia. I remember that even before pregnancy, my wife's iron levels were definitely too low. We tried to raise them with the medication prescribed by the doctor because the supplement at such a dose was not available. The levels have increased, but not enough, so my wife started eating more iron-rich products such as lean red meat, poultry, fish, eggs, groats, legumes, beets, spinach, and kale. As recently as 10-20 years ago, it was recommended to consume large amounts of iron-rich liver, but recent studies have shown that high levels of vitamin A in the liver increase the risk of fetal malformations.

Zinc has a great deal of influence on our immune system, supports growth, and improves digestion. I must point out that iron supplied to the body can reduce the absorption of zinc (yeah, I know that is paranoid!), so there should be a time gap between the consumption of products rich in these minerals.

Calcium is the building block of healthy teeth and bones. In the early stages of pregnancy (between the fourth and sixth week), the bones of the baby begin to form, so it is worth taking care to replenish the calcium before becoming pregnant.

Most of the ingredients and minerals necessary for pregnant women can be supplied with food. However, before and during pregnancy, it is recommended for women to administer foliate, one of the B vitamins that reduce the risk of a child developing neural coil defects, such as spinal fission or irreversible brain defects. Our body does not absorb folic acid from food as well as other minerals, so it is essential to supplement it. My wife also took DHA from omega-3 fatty acids. DHA plays a vital role in the development of fetal vision and brain. Taking DHA is especially noteworthy during the last trimester of pregnancy because, at that time, the brain develops at a swift pace. The acid is also good for the mother, as it reduces the risk of postpartum depression.

Now, it is worth adding a few critical facts about products that are not recommended or even prohibited and should not be consumed during pregnancy. Your partner must consume only pasteurized milk and milk products made from pasteurized milk. Special care should be taken when choosing mold and ripened cheeses as they may be contaminated with listeria, i.e., anaerobic bacteria. Despite the recommendations to consume fish, it is necessary to restrict the consumption of massive representatives of this group, such as sharks, tuna and swordfish, as they contain a lot of mercury that is toxic to the mother's body and the developing baby. Also, try to avoid raw seafood, which may cause bacterial infections or food poisoning, as well as fresh meat, eggs, and caviar, which should also be avoided due to the risk of salmonella and toxoplasmosis.

First visit to a gynecologist

Before describing the first pre-natal visit, let me point out, it is crucial to be aware of what individual medical professionals, who you may meet before and during pregnancy, are responsible for:

The GP is your first contact before any specialist appointment. He or she may send you to a midwife or refer your partner to the hospital maternity ward if the pregnancy is at increased risk. The GP may or may not prescribe the medication recommended by other specialists. If you need to use this option, remember that you will need a written recommendation from a specialist.

The midwife will be your partner's first contact. If there are any complications related to pregnancy or women's health, the midwife should inform and arrange for a consultation with the OB-GYN. Some of the midwives are educated in the environmental midwife role. They should have the necessary qualifications and skills to take care of the mother and child during pregnancy, at and after the childbirth, i.e., within six weeks after delivery.

Gynecologist - obstetrician takes care of pregnant women. Whether the pregnancy is effortless or at increased risk, the pregnant woman should be in constant contact with this doctor.

A pediatrician specializes in pediatric medicine. This is not the case in every country, but you usually choose your pediatrician on your own. You must rely on feedback from your friends or publicly available feedback, e.g., on the Internet. The pediatrician will be the primary care physician for your newborn baby.

A neonatologist is a pediatrician who specializes in neonatal medicine. Such a doctor is primarily responsible for babies with birth defects or other diseases. The neonatologist was present at the birth of my son, then he and the midwife moved by new-born son to another room. The doctor informed me about my son's health as soon as he was born and about the course of the necessary examination that they would carry out. Upon discharge from the hospital, we were advised to make an appointment with a neonatologist within about three weeks.

Nurse and midwife are primary health care for women and children. In addition to taking care during pregnancy, including performing a CT scan, the nurse[4] carries out a home visit after childbirth to check the general health of the mother and the newborn.

An anesthesiologist is a doctor specializing in anesthesiology and intensive care. His duties include administering anesthesia and pain relievers, including general anesthesia, i.e., anesthesia and local epidural or spinal anesthesia.

You are probably wondering when the first gynecologist appointment should be. There is no unambiguous answer, although it should take place between 6-8 weeks of gestation. As soon as the

---

[4]CTG is a cardiotocography, a very important test usually performed during the third trimester of pregnancy and before and during childbirth. It monitors the child's heart rate (cardiography) and records uterine contractions (tocography).

pregnancy test is positive, an appointment should be made. Of course, the date of the visit will depend on the rules in force in the specific outpatient clinic. In our case, there was no major problem because we were in the process of monitoring, i.e., we could meet with a gynecologist without a predetermined date. However, the better the specialist, the longer the waiting time for the visit. Although a private visit to our gynecologist was not the cheapest, the queue for a regular visit was about 4-5 weeks.

Here is some surprising information for you. I assume that most men (probably also women), like me, are not aware of how to calculate the week of pregnancy in which your partner is, which will undoubtedly be determined by the gynecologist at the first visit. Start your calculations by taking that pregnancy lasts for 40 weeks. Let me mention that only about 30% of all pregnancies last precisely that long. It is assumed that the properly delivered pregnancy lasts from 39 to 41 weeks. In other words, a newborn child at 39 weeks is not premature, and born at 41 weeks is not post-mature. And now this surprising piece of information: the beginning of pregnancy, that is, these 40 weeks, is not the day/night of conception, or the pregnancy test. We start counting it from the first day of the last menstrual period, so-called LMP day[5]. Why you might ask. Precisely because even when your partner is experiencing changes in her own body, and like my wife, can accurately specify the day of ovulation, she is unable to accurately determine when fertilization took place. The sperm can wait for the egg

---

[5] LMP – last menstrual period.

from 3 to 5 days after penetration into the vagina, and the egg can be fertilized within 24 hours after ovulation. It is, therefore, most natural to set the date of the first day of the last menstrual period, which is taken as the beginning of pregnancy. With a regular menstrual cycle, the first day of the last menstrual period is usually about two weeks before conception. You have probably already calculated that it will take 4 weeks (out of 40 weeks of pregnancy), and at least an additional week before the urine test will show pregnancy.

If the gynecologist of your choice had not taken care of your partner before she got pregnant, the first visit would start with an interview and a pregnancy card, which includes information about the tests carried out, their results, that is, generally speaking, the entire medical history of your partner, including the one from before pregnancy. The doctor will collect an interview about your partner's general health, lifestyle, eating habits, past, and current illnesses or medical procedures and surgeries she has undergone. You must take the pregnancy card to any scheduled doctor appointment, but it is imperative to carry it with you at all times at the later stage of pregnancy. You never know what might happen, and even if it is a minor visit to a doctor (for example, because of feeling unwell or weakening of the body), you should be able to provide all information about the pregnancy to a doctor, nurse or midwife. Create a pregnancy card folder for your partner and attach any additional results you will receive.

The first visit is an excellent opportunity for you to get answers to all the questions, so do not count on your memory to ask about everything

SOON TO BE DAD

you wanted to know and prepare notes. Whenever you have any questions or concerns, write them down on a piece of paper, phone, tablet – wherever you can. Believe me, I'm writing this from experience. If you do not write it down, in a few hours or the next day, you'll be wondering what else you should have asked. Prepare a list of questions and ask them to the doctor at the first visit.

You might want to start by asking if you should attend your partner's doctor's appointment. This is an individual matter, and it is not up to you alone. In most cases, no doctor will prohibit you from attending a visit, but this is something you need to discuss with your partner. After all, she may find herself embarrassed by your presence. We agreed that for the first few minutes of each appointment, I would wait patiently in the surgery until she finished discussing the results of the tests ordered earlier. Doctors order tests at each visit, and they are addressed in the next appointment. These are usually the results of fasting blood and urine tests. Later, the doctor performs a gynecological examination. In the first stage of pregnancy, it is often a vaginal ultrasound, during which the presence of additional people, even the closest ones, may embarrass the woman. It was only after the examination that my wife invited me in, we talked to the doctor about the current situation, and we had the opportunity to ask questions and a lot of them during each visit. At a later stage of pregnancy, the doctor performed an external ultrasound, at which I was present every time.

Pregnancy tests and examinations

At each visit, your doctor should order general blood and urine tests and ultrasound tests, the frequency of which depends on the country, the patient's state of health, or the practice used at a specific medical point. Ultrasonography is a non-invasive imaging diagnostic method. In addition to these standard tests, I present below those that can, and in some cases, must be carried out on a compulsory basis. Please note that the obligation to do so may vary from country to country:

A blood test shall be carried out:

to determine the blood type and Rh factor, anemia, and measurement of the level of the hCG hormone that I wrote about in the *Pregnancy confirmation* section. Your blood test will also tell you about your antibody levels and vitamin D levels;

to rule out hepatitis B, syphilis, chlamydias and HIV;

to detect a serological conflict that may lead to anemia in the fetus or cause jaundice and anemia in the newborn.

Cytology to rule out abnormal cells in the cervix.

Test for toxoplasmosis, a parasitic infection transmitted by animal feces, mainly cats. Recent studies estimate that around 80% of the population may be infected, but most do not realize that. If a pregnant woman becomes infected with toxoplasmosis, there is an increased chance of a miscarriage or defects in the child, manifested by blindness or mental impairment. Toxoplasmosis before pregnancy is synonymous with the acquisition of immunity and infection can only occur if the immune system is severely compromised. The disease is mainly caused by contact with cats, more specifically their feces, or by eating previously unwashed vegetables or fruit, as well as undercooked contaminated meat.

Diabetes mellitus, otherwise known as gestational diabetes mellitus - GDM, is a common complication during pregnancy and may not be related to common diabetes, although it may sometimes resemble diabetes. Pregnancy diabetes results from the enormous stress on the kidneys and the entire metabolic system of the woman. It is estimated that it affects about 2-10% of pregnant women, and almost half of women with gestational diabetes will develop type 2 diabetes within the next 15 years. One of the first studies that your doctor will or should have commissioned is glucose level test. Besides, even if the woman before pregnancy had not manifested diabetes, an analysis of the so-called sugar curve, i.e., a glucose load test, is ordered between 24 and 28 weeks of pregnancy. The test involves taking three blood samples for testing. For the first time in a fasting state. Then after drinking 75 g of glucose with water, blood is retaken for tests after the first hour and after two hours. No physical activity is allowed during the testing, as even an inconspicuous walk can affect the result. Therefore, it is best if you accompany your partner. My wife exceeded the acceptable standard in our country by only 1 mg/dl (the maximum level in our country after two hours is 199 mg/dl). In gestational diabetes, the results are zero-one analyzed. For us, this meant a visit to a diabetologist. Luckily, we ended up with a diet, not a prescription.

Prenatal screening for malformations and severe fetal diseases is a delicate topic. They are not compulsory, which is why it is up to you to decide whether or not to do so. Most babies are born healthy, but there is a risk of having a baby with a defect. The tests do not give 100% certainty, and the results indicate the probability coefficient of the defect occurrence. The birth of a disabled child may happen to anyone, but some factors are increasing the likelihood of defects. These include, but are not limited to, age over 35, previous pregnancy abnormalities, hereditary diseases in your or your partner's family.

A free fetal DNA test from the mother's blood is performed after 9 weeks of gestation when it is possible to examine the fetal DNA. It allows determining the risk of exposure to genetic diseases, including Down's syndrome. However, it is not possible to determine unequivocally whether the child is ill.

Neck translucency (NT) scan is performed at 10-13 weeks of gestation by ultrasound. It measures the distance between the skin on the neck and the subcutaneous tissue at a place called the cervical fold. This is where fluid builds up, and if there is a lot of liquid, it may mean that the child has a genetic defect, such as Down syndrome, Patau syndrome, or Edwards syndrome. There is no unambiguous answer here as to whether the child is ill or healthy, but only the probability coefficient is determined.

A **double test**, which shall be carried out in conjunction with the NT test. The combination of the results gives a more reliable answer, which is why, in our case, we decided to carry out both checks at the same time. This is a test of the concentration of two hormones: PAPP-A protein and hCG beta. A double test is performed between 10 and 14 weeks of gestation. If the combination of the double test and the NT test reveals a risk of a genetic defect, the physician should order additional tests, such as amniotic puncture and choroidal biopsy.

The **triple test** is performed at 15-20 weeks of gestation and involves the determination of three substances produced by the fetus: beta hCG, alpha-fetoprotein (AFP), and free estriol. In some countries, the inhibitor concentration is additionally determined – then we are talking **about a quadruple** test.

Ultrasound at 18-22 weeks of gestation is much more accurate than those performed during the first trimester of pregnancy. It focuses on assessing the anatomy of the fetus and identifying possible defects such as hydrocephalus, Dandy-Walker syndrome, umbilical hernia, spinal cord, cerebral or diaphragm, atresia of the small intestine or duodenum. This study will undoubtedly bring you a lot of joy because you will be able to see the developed form of your baby, i.e., the spine, legs, hands, and mouth.

Safe pregnancy

First, follow the instructions in *the section Proper diet and supplementation for the woman before and during pregnancy.* It is challenging to eliminate all threats from everyday life, but there will certainly be no problem with those which we can influence ourselves.

Smoking can inhibit fetal development, increase the risk of premature birth, or placental detachment from the uterine wall. If your pregnant partner smokes, persuade her to quit smoking, support her, and control her. If you smoke yourself, be aware that your partner's presence among smokers poses the same health risk to your child as if she smoked. If your partner can make a sacrifice, so can you.

Alcohol consumed by a woman during the first months of pregnancy may cause fetal alcohol syndrome, which in the future may cause inhibition of the growth and development of the baby or damage to the nervous system. Like smoking, alcohol harms the fetus. This is not the time for half-measures, stop drinking at all, and it is your turn to make sure the rule is followed. If your partner says that drinking small amounts of alcohol, such as a glass of wine for dinner, is not a bad thing, you need to explain to her that it hurts the developing child.

Drugs or other intoxicants also harm the child. They enter the baby's bloodstream through the placenta, increasing the risk of miscarriage. I suppose there is no need to write much about their adverse effects on the body of a woman and an unborn child.

Caffeine does not have such a detrimental effect as the drugs mentioned above. Recent research shows that supplying your body with approximately 200 mg of caffeine a day is perfectly safe for your baby. Therefore, if your partner is a coffee drinker, she does not have to give up the little black one altogether, but please note that the maximum daily amount she should not exceed is two cups or two servings of espresso.

If your partner cannot imagine a life without a **smartphone or tablet**, which is not easy these days, you can rest assured the rumors about radiation being a threat are fake news. There are no tests to confirm that. There is another reality, however. It is recommended not to wear the phone near the belly or possibly to silence it, because the fetus reacts with fear to noises, such as notification or alert sounds. Another danger is using the phone while driving. Talking or staring at your phone while walking on the street is equally dangerous. The phone could distract your partner and cause an accident.

If **your partner takes medicines**, I recommend advance contact with the doctor, and if she experiences severe pains, she should avoid aspirin, ibuprofen, and ergotamine. The safest painkiller for the pregnant is paracetamol.

Traveling during pregnancy without any contraindications to health should not cause any problems. In the case of long car journeys, ease your partner and drive. Be sure to make regular stops to stretch your legs and breathe fresh air. When fastening the seat belts, care should be taken that the lower part of the seat belt is placed under the abdomen and not on the stomach. A recommended and perfect solution is to buy or rent seat belt adapters for pregnant women. They protect the pregnant woman even better than traditional seatbelts and increase the comfort of traveling. If your partner trivializes wearing a seatbelt for discomfort, remember that professionals recommend for pregnant women to wear a seatbelt, as this increases the safety of both the mother and unborn child. Do not listen to the excuses that seatbelt compresses the uterus and disturbs the baby. The fact is that the child is surrounded by a uterine muscle wall and amniotic fluid, so it will not feel discomfort. When **traveling abroad**, be sure to check that you have current health insurance and that there are no infectious disease outbreaks in the area you are going to. And always have your pregnancy card with you.

During the "Safe Toddler" workshop in which I participated, **one of the topics was providing first aid to a pregnant woman**. If you have a general understanding of how to behave in emergencies such as choking or respiratory arrest, it is really positive. I will not describe the principles of first aid here, but I would like to quote a funny anecdote. The workshop was mainly aimed at future moms. So it was not surprising that only about 5-10% of all people were men. The lecturer (a paramedic with long experience and a father of three children) needed one man from the audience as a volunteer. Nobody was willing to help, and the confusion among the male audience was so great that I decided to help and volunteered. Behind the scenes, I was put in a tight corset with artificial women's breasts and a belly imitating the size of a woman's abdomen during the eighth month of pregnancy.

Unfortunately, I do not have any pictures, because my wife was not there in the workshop, but I must have looked ridiculous. I am quite tall and broad-shouldered, which is why the actions of a lifeguard who was at least a head shorter than me, seemed equally absurd. We set up the show backstage, and I followed paramedic's orders. One of the elements was simulating choking and presenting two grips to save me from the problem. One of the moves is to grab a woman from behind, joining hands just below her breasts. In this position, you should vigorously increase the clamp while gently lifting the entire body of the woman. You can only imagine what a well-built man dressed as a woman, and 'attacked' by a second, shorter man from behind looks like, especially when both try to jump in unison.

Cord Blood Banking

During the "Safe Toddler" workshop, I had an opportunity to listen to a representative of the stem cell bank and watch a film in which parents saved their son's life thanks to deposited blood collected at birth. Blood sampling is entirely safe for both mother and child and only takes a few minutes. You will probably ask me why we should sample blood? This blood contains stem cells that can be used to treat around 80 cancer and hematological diseases. Recent studies have shown that the administration of own cord blood has beneficial effects in the case of autism and cerebral palsy. Stem cells are also used to reconstruct neurons, joints, and bones. The collected blood can be used to treat the baby whose blood was taken at birth, as well as siblings.

The probability of stem cell treatment in the future is 1:100. So, it is entirely up to you.

Your support is essential

And that brings me to a critical point that concerns you and your commitment. As I have written before, every woman's pregnancy is different. Some feel bad, others do not notice a big difference compared to their previous well-being. It does not change the fact that a new life is developing in your partner's belly. Her system works for two, and she undoubtedly needs your support more than ever. When I write support, I mean various aspects of it, both emotional and physical, that is, your closeness and help in everyday duties.

The fact is that in many cases, the "worst" period is the first and third trimester of pregnancy. The second trimester, on the other hand, usually goes much more smoothly, and it is often the best time of the entire pregnancy. You need to get ready for your wife's nauseousness that can occur any day, any time. We, the men, may not be able to imagine this condition, but we must be aware of the hormone-induced sensitivity of pregnant women to any odors. You will probably wonder what you can do to help her with this nauseousness. You should at least try not to make her feel worse. Give up strong perfumes, which may irritate her or do not bring intensely smelling takeaway food home. Instead, buy vegetable or fruit juices and persuade her to eat five or six smaller portions spread out all over the day instead of three abundant meals. In the case of my wife, the fragrance sensitivity manifested in an incredible taste when cooking. We both love to cook, but during pregnancy, Anne outdid herself. Her dishes were always tasty, but when she was pregnant, it was just poetry.

I have only heard and read exciting stories about the wishes of pregnant women. My wife had no significant cravings and certainly did not feel like consuming any strange combinations of mismatched products. Nevertheless, you need to be prepared for this, so do not laugh at some great flavor connections. If she changes her liking and suddenly wants different foods from the ones she has eaten before, try to understand it and adapt to it. If you like varied cuisine, you will probably not mind being sent to buy a chocolate pizza instead of chicken.

Be prepared for your partner's mood swings. The good news is that they may mainly be intensified in the first trimester when hormone levels change rapidly. Unfortunately, this emotional swing can accompany a woman until and even after childbirth. This is why you will need some angelic patience. Halt your emotions, weigh the words, and always try to relieve tension so that there is no quarrel. What else can you do? If she gets depressed, offer a snack to raise her glucose. If you never went for walks before, this is a good time for a change. Walking is a form of physical activity, and each exercise releases endorphins, the hormones of happiness.

Strengthen the bond with your partner. Talk about everything, which concerns you both and your child. You must be aware that pregnancy is the most important thing to her right now, and your position at home might be less central. Turning things around like this can make you feel rejected, but remember, it is only temporary. Conversation and spending time together will undoubtedly strengthen your relationship. Establish an emotional bond with your unborn child, talk to him, stroke your wife's tummy. This may seem ridiculous to you, but remember, your child can hear you and may recognize your voice. The child will also know your voice as soon as it is born, which will make it feel safe in your arms. A close relationship with your partner might be created by your participation in medical examinations, so if you have an opportunity, do not have second thoughts. I particularly remember my commitment during pregnancy. Frankly speaking, this engagement still has not passed away, although today it is focussed at my son. I remember the smile on the neonatologist's face during our son's first visit. She addressed concrete questions to my wife (Which pregnancy is it? In which week was the baby born? Was the delivery natural or cesarean? What was the birth weight? What was the position of the child?), but she did not have a chance to answer, as I volunteered to comment on these points before her.

Do not get angry when your partner cannot sleep at night. Insomnia is a natural symptom of pregnancy. Her body is freaking out because some individual entity is growing in it. In the third trimester, difficulty sleeping or light sleep is caused by an increase in the abdomen, which causes discomfort. The best position is the side position. Special pillows for pregnant women are beneficial here, as they help to get comfortable in bed on the one hand and serve as an indispensable gadget when feeding the baby on the other. If her insomnia keeps you up, do not get nervous, try to socialize instead. Serve warm tea or milk if she feels like drinking. Offer a massage or prepare a hot bath.

If your partner gave up alcohol during pregnancy. This is great! Support her and make her feel like she is not alone. Give up drinking for that time as well. I did so. You can find more details on it in the last chapter, *Child as the best motivator*. What, I am sure your partner will appreciate is taking over her chores on a day-to-day basis. It all depends on how your responsibilities were shared between you so far. Remember, even though she does not seem to do anything, she may feel tired as she lives and works for two. Try to make her life more comfortable, clean the apartment, do the laundry, put the clothes away, take care of dinner, unload the dishwasher.

Sign up with your partner for a birth course. At the birth school, not only do they prepare the woman for childbirth, but they also focus on the time of delivery (the first six weeks after childbirth), including the care of the newborn. Think of it as a source of knowledge. I'm sure you will not regret your participation, and your partner may feel that you support her and that you want to prepare well for the role of the daddy.

If you can be there for her during childbirth, do it. She will surely need it so much. You have to be a paragon of restraint and keep calm. Especially if it is the first delivery. She does not know what to expect (neither do you). In the initial phase, ensure peace and make her comfortable. Talk to her to distract her. At this stage, contractions are not so frequent yet, so do not lose your temper and do not let her lose hers. In the next steps of childbirth, lift her spirits all the time, try to be her contact with hospital staff, remind her about the toilet, suggest a change of position, massage her neck, hold her hand. Tell the nurse or doctor if contractions get worse and more frequent. If cervical dilation is significant, it may be the last stage of labor.

Couvade syndrome, or male sympathetic pregnancy

Are you pregnant, too? Well, if you are reading this guidebook, you are undoubtedly involved in your partner's pregnancy. Some men engage so much that they may experience some of the symptoms experienced by a pregnant woman. According to a study by a team of scientists at St. George's University in London, sympathetic pregnancy is an increasingly common phenomenon. It turned out that the examined men felt so much sympathy for the condition of their partners that they were not only affected by mood changes or insomnia but also nausea, cravings, and back pain. Symptoms may also include vomiting, constipation, tiredness, muscle spasms, dizziness, and even weight gain. The latter does not surprise me at all, because, from the observation of my friends who were expecting a child, I can conclude that this is a fairly common condition.

Around 80% of future fathers share the feeling of being pregnant, 75% have food cravings and appetites, half of them notice mood swings, and one in five feel postpartum depression. What can you do about it? Use the information provided in the last chapter, *Child as the best motivator*. Setting goals and making changes in your life will help you reduce stress and kill time to such an extent that sympathetic pregnancy symptoms will decrease. If you do not have similar symptoms, do not worry, it does not mean that you are not committed enough to your partner's pregnancy or that you are not ready to be a dad.

If you would like to know more check my book ***"Couvade Syndrome: What Male Sympathetic Pregnancy is & how you can Fight it"*** **(ASIN: B086ZZK2XC).**

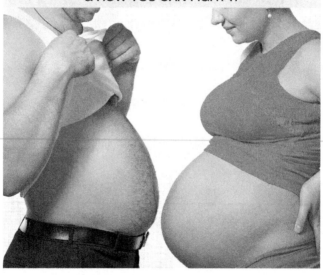

PREPARATION FOR THE CHILDBIRTH

You must be excited to be a future dad, right? I am also sure that at the back of your head, you have some paternity issues, and you are wondering how you are going to handle it. Well, you have already taken the first step in seeking information when reaching for this guide. Remember, neither of us is born a father. Parenting comes naturally. That's how nature made us.

On the third day after the birth of our son, while we were still in the hospital, we ran into a young and brilliant neonatologist, whom I asked to come to our room to discuss some specific issues related to the harmless procedure she was to perform for our son. I was impressed with the doctor's attitude towards children. I wish you could find an equally excellent doctor. She shared with us a lot of valuable hints, including tips on breastfeeding and lifting and holding the baby. We always heard of the need to support the head as a little man cannot keep it straight. She grabbed our baby boy with one hand placed under his chest, lifted him up, and, helping herself with the other hand, began to gently rotate his body in such a way that the head started to revolve around the body and the child took the embryonic position. We make similar movements when shaking head during the warm-up or stretching cervical vertebrae. At first, I was a little scared, and I even thought she might harm my son. But after a while, I realized that she grabbed him in such a delicate way that she could not hurt him. Then she said: *Do not listen to everything your grandmothers tell you, do not read advice on Internet forums, get carried away by nature and maternal instincts. The hare carries his little ones by the sticking ears, the cat runs with the little ones holding them by the neck. Their cubs hang inert, and they are not harmed, because it is all-natural.* So remember – get carried away by nature!

You all know, you have a lot of errands to run before the baby is born. I am not going to tell you, you are wrong. Frankly speaking, just because I have such a consistent wife, we managed to get it all together in time. Let's face it, shopping for clothes is not a man's business, although nothing is embarrassing about it if you are the one who has to take care of it. I was wondering where my wife got her knowledge of things that she needed to buy. It is not like she read the same books I did. And even if she did, there was no exact information about it. I think it was the abundance of information found on the Internet. However, the most important source of information was friends who had given birth, those who were pregnant, or who planned to get pregnant. If you want, you can buy clothes yourself, but I am sure your partner will have a better sense of style and, most importantly, a sense of size. You will probably notice that each brand, and even products of the same brand, despite the same size numbering, differ in size. Buying clothes will bring a lot of joy to your partner, so do not try to deprive her of it.

However, she probably will not let you do it. I remember buying the first fleece romper for my unborn son. It felt fantastic. Now, writing this sentence, our son is out of the bath, and he has precisely this romper I bought for him. On this occasion, I would like to mention that the very first purchase for my son was disposable diapers. I was incredibly excited about this purchase, I felt enormous satisfaction, and yet these were just diapers. I was waiting proudly in line, thinking that the saleswoman, would see my purchase, and ask me about the baby, and I would proudly say that I would soon become a father. She did not ask.

Back to shopping planning, I'm not suggesting that you do exactly what I do, but an excellent way to start is to make a list of things to do and all the necessary products you should stock up on. When you're expecting a baby, you become a kind of shopaholic, and you may find yourself buying either too much or unnecessary things. Not all the items on the list can be purchased in one store or, if they are available, prices might vary considerably. However, if the price is a secondary issue, I see no reason why you should not buy most of the stuff in one or two places. We decided to use online shopping from two or three vendors. Of course, for some products, it is better to go and see them live to evaluate quality. But let's face it, in the age of developed online sales and no need to justify returns of goods, online shopping is very convenient. Just remember not to put it off for the last minute. I know from experience I could have handled a few things much earlier, although we dealt with the most important ones well in advance.

I have already mentioned that we approach everything with common sense and do not make essential decisions spontaneously. In the case of strategic purchases, such as a stroller or a car seat, we had serious discussions for a very long time to properly use this considerable amount of money. Keep in mind that in case of most accessories you buy, your child's safety comes first. You need to be sure of your choice, and in particular not to make emotional decisions, such as in-store decisions. Following the instigation of a smart salesman who knows how to sell everything is also not very sensible. Trust me, they can sell even the most worthless products. In the following sections, I will tell you what to pay attention to when choosing products for your baby to make you both happy.

The place for a child

This is undoubtedly one of the first things you need to think about when planning or waiting for a child. Bed space, changing table, wardrobe or clothing shelf, handy place for cosmetics, organizers, diapers, and other accessories - you need to think about all this and organize the space in the child's room very well. If you do not yet have an apartment large enough for a child to have its own separate room, or if you simply want the child to share a place with you for the first period of his or her life, you have to prepare and plan enough space. In our case, we already knew a few years before birth that we would be trying to have a baby, so we took this into account when renovating our bedroom and changing furniture.

Furniture, cot, mattress

When planning the new bedroom furniture, we decided to leave room for a standard size cot, right next to the furniture built precisely according to our own idea. Together with the furniture producing craftsman, we employed a smart design. We did it in such a way that the baby cot was right next to the wardrobe with baby clothes, which in the first months, and perhaps even years, would most often be used, i.e., bodysuits and rompers. Of course, the clothes we use now are so small that folded in half, they can be arranged in drawers vertically. Now, when choosing the right clothes, we select them as if they were files in a drawer. Other cabinets and shelves are used for storing larger clothes, including outer clothing and blankets, towels, tetra diapers (irreplaceable parental gadget).

The cot has standard dimensions (47x23 inch), although, of course, you can find both larger and smaller ones. The most popular are those made of pinewood; however, this is not the rule. There are countless decorations available, but, just like in the case of colors, it is a matter of taste. What you should pay attention to, apart from visual considerations, is the possibility of adjusting the level of the mattress base. You can then lower it as the child grows and starts crawling or standing. In our cot bed, you can additionally remove the three front bars, which gives you a smart opening. A walking toddler can use it to enter or leave the cot bed by himself, and while sleeping and playing, the other bars still keep him safe. The spacing between the bars must not exceed 6 cm. If you do not have a lot of space, it would be good if the cot was equipped with an additional drawer where you can store small things, such as diapers, cotton swabs, tissues, base sheets, etc. Remember not to put any stuffed animals or blankets in the cot as they pose a danger of suffocation.

Another item you need to purchase to complete your child's cot bed is a **mattress**. It seems like such a trivial matter, and yet choosing the right mattress did not come easy to us. Start by checking if the mattress has the necessary approvals and certificates to confirm the absence of hazardous chemicals. Consider that the baby will spend a lot of time in the cot while its entire skeletal system will be shaping and developing. We began to explore the subject and read the opinions of physiotherapists. Imagine an infant who has not yet developed motor coordination and whose muscles are weak. Do not make it harder for him to move by buying an overly soft mattress. A soft mattress can also make it difficult to turn the head or try to lift while lying on the tummy and trying to raise clumsily on the hands. Focus on medium-hard mattresses so the child's spine can shape adequately.

OK, so the hardness is checked. What about the filling of the mattress? The market offers quite a lot of possibilities:

Foam mattress - consists entirely of foam, or it can be a combination of different types of foam at the same time. Yes, there are various types of foam available. Some are better and some worse. The foam mattress is quite popular; therefore it is necessary to go into the specification of the material it is made of:

polyurethane foam which is susceptible to deformation and rapidly loses its elasticity;

highly flexible polyurethane foam, also referred to as HR, is much more durable and has excellent flexibility and elasticity – it is a perfect choice for the newborn and infant;

thermoplastic foam behaves very similar to HR foam. Influenced by temperature, it adapts to the baby's body, but it has a disadvantage of accumulating heat, which can lead to overheating the baby.

Spring mattress - as the name suggests, there are springs inside, while the outer sides are usually made of foam. These mattresses are very comfortable, however, due to the low weight of the child, the correct operation of such a mattress cannot be achieved. This filling is worth considering in the case of a few years old children.

Latex mattress – manufacturers boast that they are anti-allergic and anti-bacterial, but the truth is entirely different. The proteins contained in latex may cause allergic reactions. Instead, we can use actually-allergenic synthetic latex, but it will not be characterized by breathability, as is the case of natural latex.

Coconut buckwheat mattress - the insert is made of natural coconut fibers, while the other side consists of buckwheat. Such a mattress is very airy, and buckwheat adapts to the body, so it is recommended that the infant sleeps on the coconut side during the first few months of life. You need to make sure if the mattress has the necessary approvals to eliminate the possibility of using buckwheat from crops where chemicals have been used. Recently, however, there has been some controversial news on natural buckwheat or coconut inserts. As they are susceptible to moisture absorption, they might cause mold growth.

Other combined mattresses – there are many different combinations of layers, e.g., foam+buckwheat or buckwheat+coconut+foam.

Baby stroller

Besides the car seat, the stroller is one of the most expensive products you need to buy, so do not take this decision without proper consideration. A well-chosen stroller will make life easier for you and your partner. The offer on the market is enormous. Apart from various shapes and colors, there are many types of strollers: full-sized strollers, also known as prams, light-weight or umbrella strollers, multi-functional, or even jogging strollers. Make a list or define points that would characterize a stroller to meet your expectations. Currently, the most popular strollers are:

A deep stroller also referred to as 2-in-1. It consists of a chassis, bassinet, and the convertible attached stroller seat mounted on the same frame. For about the first six months, when the baby still does not sit up, you can use a bassinet attached to the chassis. In the bassinet, the child travels in a lying position. As soon as it begins to sit up, you need to detach the bassinet and attach the seat of the stroller. This kind of stroller can be used from birth to the moment the child starts walking. 2-in-1 seems to be one of the best choices.

Multi-functional stroller also referred to as 3-in-1. This set includes a chassis, bassinet, stroller seat, and a chassis-compatible car seat. This stroller is very versatile, but it also has its drawbacks. It is often heavy and non-reversible. If your choice is this type of stroller, pay special attention to the car seat included in the set. It is often the case that the seat itself is not as robust and safe as the car-seat purchased separately. It may also not have the necessary approvals and certifications, which is the topic of the next section.

Light-weight stroller also referred to as an umbrella. This is a typical stroller that you will start using as soon as the baby begins to sit. Unlike the 2-in-1 or 3-in-1 stroller sitting conversion, the umbrella is a light and handy stroller. Once folded like an umbrella, it takes up very little space, so it can be easily transported or stored.

Each of these strollers should be equipped with additional accessories such as rain foil, bassinet cover, bassinet mattress, care bag with chassis handle attachment, bottom luggage compartment, i.e., a handy pocket to take the necessary items or shopping.

For us, additional details were essential. Our baby's ultrasound showed he was going to be a big boy. All indicators (femur length, abdomen, and head circumference) were within the normal range, but above average, which is why we prepared for a large (read, long) child. Therefore, the internal length of the bassinet and the height of the stroller seat backrest were essential for us. Another vital element was the chassis, which is why when comparing several models of strollers, I was interested in the weight and dimensions of the folded frame so that it did not take up a lot of space in the trunk of the car. The other aspects we highlighted were the shock absorber system, the wheels (inflatable or full rubber), the brake that can be released using the sole of the shoe (in most strollers, the brake is released using the upper part of the foot, which can easily damage the leather shoes), the overall ease of ride, the appearance, and available colors.

I encourage you to visit several stores and talk to the sellers. Just do not let them tell you into buying it right away. Consider the seller as a source of information at this stage. Do not be discouraged if you run into a seller who does not impress you with knowledge. I visited three large stores with a similar assortment, and only in two stores, I found the right, competent people.

Child safety seat

The offered range of child safety seats is as wide as the offer of strollers. Until your child no longer needs to use a car seat, you will have to use three types of car seats. In this guide, I am going to focus on the first child safety seat you are going to use for about a year.

The obligation to use child car-seat while driving is regulated by the law, but the most important thing for you is that it guarantees the highest possible level of safety for your child. It is becoming an increasingly common practice in hospitals to prevent parents from taking a child home unless they can show they are going to use the right car-seat. Please note that the regulations governing the use of car seats may differ from country to country.

Each commercially available seat shall be appropriately approved and certified, which is confirmed by a sticker, generally affixed to the underside of the chair. Approvals vary depending on the part of the world. Currently, there are two standards in force in the European Union: the older one – ECE R44-04 (equivalent to FMVSS 213 in the USA and RSSR in Canada) and the newer ECE R129 referred to as i-Size. To be approved to ECE R44-04, seats shall be tested in frontal collisions between vehicles at 50 km/h and rear collisions at the speed of 30 km/h. The results are provided by dummies placed in seats and attached to sensors. The i-Size approval, which applies in parallel, is the result of establishing a special UN commission, which defined more advanced safety criteria in 2013, including the seat side-impact tests. The i-Size introduces a seat fit based on the child's age and height, not weight. Seats are additionally tested by independent organizations. In Germany, it is ADAC, in the UK – AA, in Austria - OEAMTC, in the USA – NHTSA.

All i-Size seats and the vast majority of 'old' type approval seats are compatible with the ISOFIX system available in cars. This is a system of two handles located between the backrest and the rear seat of the vehicle and attached directly to the vehicle structure. In the case of a newborn child seat, to use the ISOFIX system, you must purchase the so-called seat base, which you need to attach to the ISOFIX handles. The base has its pros and cons. It is very comfortable to use because we can easily connect a seat to it literally in seconds. The base reflects the safety of the car seat mounting, so we do not have to worry that anything went wrong when putting the child's car seat into the car. The base will typically be compatible with the next car seat you buy if you limit yourself to the same manufacturer, as other brands' bases and car seats are usually not compatible with each other. An additional downside is a price. Often, the base costs as much as the car-seat.

The other way to secure the child car seat is to use standard belts (without the base for attaching ISOFIX). The lower lap straps shall pass through the buckles in the lower part of the seat and the upper part through the buckle on its back. To secure and tighten the seat belts correctly, it is best to push the seat back into the car seat and tighten the seat belts.

What else should you pay attention to? Inserts to stabilize the baby in the car seat are also crucial. Some models let you pull out even two inserts. This allows the child seat to be correctly adjusted to the size (or preferably width) of the child. Please note that a child wearing a jumpsuit in winter will need more space. Some models have fixed-mounted inserts, but you can also find seats with additional side inserts, which you can pull out if necessary to increase the seat space. Make sure the inserts are profiled to protect the baby's neck and head from excessive sideways movement. According to the latest findings, the seat cushion should be at an angle of 45-50 degrees. This is the safest position for the infant. Note that the rear seats of the vehicle where the child car-seat is mounted can be placed at different angles depending on the car model. This is why you should go to the store before buying, and ask for the seat to be placed in the car, and then check the final angle of the car seat. You can do this by downloading a smartphone app, which, when you put it on the seat cushion, checks the angle of inclination.

Here, I can add another fascinating insight, which is not widely known, and about which the physiotherapist involved in designing the car seat I chose told me (yes, I managed to reach him when I tried to talk to the manufacturer on the phone to explain inaccuracies in the product description on the website). Most infant seats are designed in such a way that the position of the toddler is somewhat sitting position, which negatively affects the not yet fully-formed spine. A massive head falls forward down, and the toddler cannot lift it. This causes bending in the neck section, thus making breathing difficult. Only a few manufacturers pay attention to this at the design stage, and from the full market offer, I found only two seats of different brands that guaranteed a better position for the infant, i.e., more lying than a sitting position.

Also, keep in mind that wherever there is right-hand traffic, you should place a seat at the back right. In the event of a breakdown, collision, accident, or traffic jam, this site will not endanger your health or life while pulling the baby out of the car. Encourage your partner not to sit in the back with the child while traveling, as the safest place for her is the front passenger seat. Imagine what could happen in an accident when your partner would take care of the baby while riding at the backseat and not wearing her seat belt, as it happens all the time.

She could put herself and the baby at risk. And mind you, we always mount the seat backward.

Baby Clothes

This section should be at the very beginning because I am sure that baby clothes will be one of the first, if not the first, things you buy. Despite trying to refrain yourselves from buying excess garments, you will still buy more than enough. A newborn grows on a week to week basis (or even day to day), so keep it on your mind when purchasing another cute romper. In the first weeks and months, the best clothes will be rompers, one-piece overalls with long legs and sleeves, and bodysuits, i.e., crotch snap-fastened shirts. Depending on the season and current weather, long-sleeved and short-sleeved bodysuits are the best. The most convenient are those with a slit in the front and a snap-fastening on the side. It is also referred to as an envelope fastening. Most rompers and sleeping shirts are sewn with feet that provide warmth, and thus, do not require socks. Sometimes we put extra socks on these feet anyway, although you have to remember that the baby may have cold hands and feet, which does not indicate that he or she is cold. Body temperature is best checked on the baby's neck.

When it comes to two-piece outfits, they look impressive but are not as practical as one-piece rompers. However, the fact remains, it is good to purchase at least some of such sets. You can choose from tracksuits, as well as sweatpants and sweater combinations. These are fantastic garments to use as a festive outfit. Besides, it is excellent to buy a few pairs of socks and hats. The light ones are, for instance, the best after a bath.

Of course, it is also essential to think of outerwear, which largely depends on seasons. For the autumn-winter season, overalls with gloves, scarf, and a thicker hat would be indispensable. Buying overalls, avoid those with slippery materials on the outside. You will appreciate this hint when putting the baby into the car seat. The list of clothes you need to take to the hospital can be found in the section *Hospital layette*.

Baby's first aid kit and care supplies

In the home first aid kit, or more specifically, your child's first aid kit, there should be the following items:

Painkiller and antipyretic based on paracetamol and/or ibuprofen. Remember, however, that ibuprofen-based medicines should be used from the age of three months. Baby painkillers are available in two forms: liquid or suppositories. Also remember, aspirin must not be given to infants or children under 12 years of age. You may ask why. Aspirin contains acetylsalicylic acid, which can cause Reye's syndrome, a disease that rarely occurs but is life-threatening.

Wound disinfectant, e.g., Octenisept, which is also recommended for the daily care of the umbilical cord stump before it falls off after about 7-14 days.

Irrigant and electrolyte replenishment fluids to help with the baby's diarrhea.

An antibiotic ointment prescribed by your doctor for scratches and minor cuts.

Sea salt for the nose – used as a spray to care for the child's nose, i.e., to relieve runny nose problems or infections of the upper respiratory tract.

An **infant nasal bulb or nasal aspirator**, which, combined with sea salt, will provide help with your baby's nose. Personally, I use a nasal aspirator (connected to a vacuum cleaner), which despite my previous concerns, is very safe. My son likes to clean his nose that way – it always calms him down.

Sterile swabs will be helpful, e.g., for daily eye care with **saline**.

Thermometer - there are many different types of thermometers (rectal, auricular, temporal, oral), but experts agree that the most reliable result is rectal temperature checking.

Other products that you can supply the baby's first aid kit with are: adhesive bandages, tweezers, nail scissors, insect bite and itchy rash preparation, ointment for nappy rashes, hot water bag.

Supply the baby first aid kit with care supplies:

Bath Liquid/Gel – choose those for infants as they have a mild composition.

Baby Care Oil - choose those intended for infants, because they differ in composition, among others, they are not fragrant. Recently, there are more and more opponents of using baby care oils because, despite initial lubrication, they can dry the skin.

Face cream for babies.

Face cream, which protects against cold and wind – the best choice is the cream, which does not contain water.

Sunscreen – remember to protect the baby from prolonged sunlight exposure, despite the use of sunscreen.

Comb and/or hairbrush - it is best to use a natural bristle brush for everyday care, while backcombing and moisturizing, e.g., with baby care oil, is recommended in the event of ecchymosis, in other words, peeling of the scalp.

Feeding accessories

The list of feeding products will depend on whether your partner uses breastfeeding or bottle-feeding (or both). If it is breast food you use, you don't really need anything, except for an element that can make it easier to position the baby and lighten your partner's burden, which might be a feeding pillow. In addition to feeding, such pillows help pregnant women find a comfortable sleeping position.

For emergency feeding or bottle feeding, you should purchase the following accessories:

Babies' feeding bottles There is a vast selection of these items, so choose those without BPA (bisphenol A), a chemical present in many plastic products. BPA is suspected of damaging the nervous system, disrupting hormones, and increasing the risk of heart disease. Studies in the US show that as many as 90% of Americans are found to have BPA in their urine. The US Food and Drug Administration and the European Commission have banned the production of cups and bottles for infants and children using BPA. Manufacturers brag on the labels of their products about the lack of BPA in production, but this should be approached with caution as they use BPS (bisphenol S), which can have a similar effect on the body as BPA.

You can choose from all sorts of bottles, e.g., classic, anti-colic, orthodontic, bleeder bottles. You have to test for yourself which bottle and pacifier best fit your baby.

The bottle dryer is a brilliant product in its simplicity. Even if you use a dishwasher, you'll need a small dryer where you can put away your washed bottles and pacifiers.

A breast pump will be needed if your partner wants to breastfeed in case of excess breast milk, or if, as in our case, she will try to evoke breastfeeding in the first days or weeks after giving birth. You can choose a manual or electric breast pump. We used an electric one, first a single one (for one breast), then a double one (for two breasts at the same time), which shortened the extraction time.

Food storage containers are essential if you are going to freeze milk or store it briefly in a refrigerator. Breast milk can be kept at room temperature for up to 8 hours and refrigerated for 2 to 4 days.

Thermos – for storing hot water when you are away from home, and your partner is not with you.

Powdered milk container – preferably one with separate chambers, where you can put measured portions. Ideal when you are away from home without your partner.

A device for heating bottles and jars. The one I use has an additional bottle sterilization function.

A pacifier that, while not used for feeding, will satisfy your baby's need for sucking between meals.

Other accessories

Changing table – it is worth using until the baby grows up, and you can change it elsewhere. It is usually covered with waterproof material. Changing table covers/sheets are also available for purchase. Remember not to leave the baby unattended on the changing table.

Cot organizer - there are many types of organizers you can attach to the cot. I picked one with a lot of pockets. It allows me to have everything at my fingertips when I am changing or nursing my son on the changing table.

Closet and drawer organizers - will help you store and access clothes or small accessories quickly.

Diapers – whether non-disposable or disposable, you can't do without them. I am not suggesting what to use – you are to decide. I use disposable ones, and I can tell you that in the first few weeks, with frequent poops, a whole bunch of them is used. Approximately after 6 weeks, the digestive system stabilizes, and defecation frequency decreases. Do not be surprised if there is only one XXL size poop in 1-2 days.

Dirty diaper container – it is good to have a small box where, after changing the baby, you can throw dirty diapers.

Moisturized wipes - they are cheap and convenient, helpful when wiping a dirty fanny while changing diapers. However, recent studies have shown that the ingredients contained in them are harmful to the youngest and exacerbate the symptoms of skin diseases. At home, I use **cosmetic pads** dipped in lukewarm water, and moisturized wipes when I am away from home.

Draw-sheets – I use them additionally on a changing pad covered with sheets. It is easier to replace the soiled draw-sheet than to wash the cloth sheet every time. The draw-sheets come in different sizes, I use 23"x15". They work equally well if you are changing the baby in a different place than the changing table or when you are away.

Tetra, flannel or muslin diapers – they act as cloths and pose indispensable gadget for a young parent. They are suitable for wiping the baby's mouth when it spits up or as a draw-sheet when you are away from home.

Mattress sheet in a cot - although the mattress cover can be washed, it is easier to clean the cloth. Some people also use waterproof draw-sheets, but they are also air-tight, so in my opinion, they are useless.

Portable/hiking bed - this is an option for a regular cot. A portable baby bed can be attached to your bed so that you have a baby at your fingertips. They are foldable, so you can take them on holiday, for instance.

Baby bouncer – it works great when the child is awake, and you have some household chores that you need to use two hands for. You can then put the baby bouncer in the room where you are, and keep an eye on the junior. Some baby bouncers have extra vibrations or tunes to calm the baby down.

Swaddle wrap – it is worth to purchase at least one. If you cannot wrap the baby in a blanket, so it does not get out of the cocoon, the swaddle wrap will be beneficial. A baby wrapped in a blanket in a so-called envelope or placed in a swaddle wrap feels very safe. It's warm and tight, almost like his mother's tummy.

Blankets – if you can wrap a swaddle, you can use the blanket right away. If you cannot, you'll need it soon. You can put the blanket on the bed to put the baby on it, cover the baby in the stroller while walking on colder days, or use it to cover the baby in the cot when junior no longer wants to sleep in a swaddle wrap or cocoon. Caution, due to the risk of so-called cot death or sudden infant death syndrome - SIDS (in this case by uncontrolled choking with a blanket), it is not recommended to cover sleeping children with a blanket. As early as 3-4 weeks old, my son began to prefer blanket cover, but at the same time, he did not like to be covered up to the neck, so the upper edge of the blanket was always under his armpits, limiting the possibility of putting the blanket on his face in an uncontrollable way.

Sleeping bag – an alternative to a swaddle wraps and blankets. Besides, the swaddle wrap, this is the safest way to keep the baby warm without the risk of SIDS.

Rattles/mascots - as soon as the little one starts focusing eyes, small mascots are an excellent idea to arouse the interest. Choose the ones with bright colors that will attract the child's attention. Over time, they will help with grip exercises. You can also buy small mascots with Velcro attachment for hands or feet.

Bathtub – small plastic baths are great when bathing a baby. There is a vast selection of colors and patterns, some of which have thermometers glued inside. However, a thermometer is not needed to test the temperature of the water. Your elbow immersed in the water is the best sensor.

Bath towels - these baby towels have a double corner where you can put the baby's wet head after the bath.

Stroller sleeping bag – useful for colder days. You can use it both in the bassinet as well as in the stroller or even on the sled. Make a note of the holes through which you can pass the seat belts.

Laundry detergents – do not take risks and choose only those for babies. Why is that? These for adults contain detergents that can cause allergies or irritation, and the skin of young children is susceptible.

Hospital layette

I know there are a lot of essential things to take care of before the birth of a child. However, you cannot forget to prepare the hospital layette for the infant and the mother. I decided to devote a separate section to this list. Remember not to put it off until the last minute. It will save you a lot of stress right before the birth, and get you prepared, in case the little one decides to come into this world a bit faster. And the most important - I know it from experience. Medical care is different in every country. There are countries where you do not even have to bring baby clothes with you because you get them on the spot. The list below contains all the things you need, assuming you have to take care of whatever it takes.

Mom's bag:

✓ Documents and test results, i.e., pregnancy card with medical test results. It is best to keep the whole file in one folder, which should be taken to each doctor's appointment and for further trips, as I elaborated on it in the *Safe pregnancy* section;

✓ identity card and insurance;

✓ medicines if your partner is taking any;

✓ long cotton T-shirts for childbirth 1-2pk;

✓ single-use panties, several pieces;

✓ feeding bras 2pk;

✓ unbuttoned nightdresses (for feeding) 2pk;

✓ socks, several pairs;

✓ bathrobe;

✓ a zipper sweatshirt;

✓ clean clothes for hospital discharge;

✓ slippers, shower flip flops;

✓ cord blood collection kit, if you use this option;

✓ hygiene and cosmetic products: deodorant, toothpaste and toothbrush, soap, shower gel, hair shampoo, intimate hygiene liquid, comb or brush, towels (2pk including small towel), disposable tissues, liners and overnight pads, lactation pads, paper towel;

✓ foodstuffs: still water, juices (citrus are not recommended), biscuits, crackers;

✓ notebook and pen.

Child's bag:

✓ jammies, 3pk;

✓ shirts/child's vests 3pk;

✓ bodysuits, 3pk;

✓ infant hats/caps 2pk;

✓ socks;

✓ blanket;

✓ swaddle wrap;

✓ disposable or reusable diapers;

✓ tetra/flannel/muslin napkins (serving as tissues);

✓ bath towel;

✓ neonatal bath fluid;

✓ evaporation cream;

✓ moisturized wipes;

✓ hygiene pads;

✓ clothes for hospital discharge depending on the season.

CHILD IS THE BEST MOTIVATOR

Waiting for a child is the perfect time to make a difference in your life. I dare to write this – it may be the last chance for a change. No New Year's resolution will motivate you to make changes in your life the way an unborn child can. Whether you are going to quit smoking, alcohol, gain weight or lose weight, learn a foreign language, learn salsa or complete a welder course, I know from personal experience that this is not easy, but I can also confirm that if your child is the motivator of these changes, you will not give up and do your job. At the end of this guide, I'd like to tell you my story. It might inspire you to make your own choices.

I am not the one to keep the resolutions, although I must admit that about seven years ago, I noticed that my weight was too high. Looking at the pictures from those years now, I wonder how I got into this mess. At that time, I decided to invest in a balanced diet created by a specialist, which did not involve many sacrifices. I always thought hunger was something natural when trying to lose weight. But that was not the case. Within about 11 months, I lost 50 pounds, which I thought was a huge personal success. The big problem is the so-called yo-yo effect, i.e., the return to the same or higher weight than before the diet. In my case, there was no such effect because, with the menu, I changed my eating habits, and I still stick to it today. I may sometimes turn a blind eye and eat something unhealthy or miss one workout, but we are not robots, right?

I mentioned the male sympathetic pregnancy earlier. I am not sure, but it seems this phenomenon is the only reason future fathers and young fathers put on weight. I noticed this among my friends. What happens to us, men, when waiting for a child? How come waiting for a kid or a small child at home changes our behavior to the point that we get fat? I have a theory based on my experience, which I will refer to later in this story.

Being aware of the risk that I might look the same, the moment I found out we were expecting a baby, I told myself that I cannot be like other people, i.e., young fathers with large bellies. The goal I set was not only to maintain weight but to completely get rid of my slightly imperfect belly and generally improve my body build and fitness. I pictured myself in the future, jogging with my teenage son, who caught up my healthy lifestyle. Given the above, I introduced regular exercises six times a week. Three times a week, I went to a gym, where I did not focus on aerobics, but rather exercised strength, and then I jogged three times a week. I went jogging, although I did not like it at first. To be honest, I did not like long-distance running since I was a kid. I could run 65 yd or 110 yd sprints, but long-distance runs made me tired. Of course, the first time I tried jogging, I thought I would run my lungs out. My fitness was terrible. I had a lot of moments of weakness when I wanted to give up, but that is when I always thought about my unborn baby and that I have to overcome this for him because he is the reason I am doing it.

I started with three or 1.5 to 2.5-mile joggings. It is quite natural that in the beginning, it was a jog mixed with march and jogtrot. However, over time, as the muscles strengthened and my fitness level improved, I started to jog at a 3-mile distance without any breaks. Over time, I increased the range, mainly at weekends, until I reached 7.5 or even 8 miles, which was a massive success for me. At the very beginning of my running career, I set myself the goal of participating and completing some running competition. When I could run the maximum distance of about 3-3.5 miles, I registered for the 6-mile run, and then I had no choice. All right, I could have backed out, but I was doing it for my son, I mean, I wanted to be able to brag that I was working on my fitness at the time and finished this run for him. In fact, I completed the cross-country race with a large number of hills at a distance of 6.5 miles in 1:06 h. If you jog regularly, you are probably not impressed by this result, but I am proud of myself because I kept my resolution despite the temptation to let it go. In moments of weakness, even when I was jogging, I thought about my son, and I did not give up.

What is the effect of this physical activity? I love running. You can really get addicted to it. My physical strength, fitness, and general well-being have improved. It is normal that after physical exercise, endorphins called hormones of happiness are secreted, but general well-being stays with you in your daily life. Did I lose weight? As a matter of fact, I can surprise you. I did not lose weight; well, all in all, I lost maybe 4 pounds. But I was amazed because people who met me and whom I had not seen for a few months immediately said that I had lost weight. I felt that I was losing weight, but in my case, the jogging combined with a balanced diet and exercise made me lose fat tissue while developing muscles at the same time. Therefore, I can say that my body build looks much better than before my wife got pregnant. I am generally pleased and proud of myself, but I only owe it to the motivation I gained in thinking about my son and that I was doing it all for him. Remember, do not make excuses when making changes. You will probably say you do not have time. Well, everyone has the same amount of time. I did not want to devote my afternoons to physical activity, either. After all, we all have responsibilities. So what did I do? I got up an hour early and ran before work. After work, I could enjoy my afternoon, just like before I started training.

I did not limit my resolutions solely to the struggle for my own body and fitness. I gave up drinking alcohol at all during pregnancy. This way, I expressed solidarity with my wife, who had to give up the glass of wine that we enjoyed at weekends for the time of pregnancy (and breastfeeding). On the one hand, I wanted my wife to feel my support, on the other hand, I always remembered that I was doing it for my son.

I would like to go back to my theory about male sympathetic pregnancy and one of its effects, i.e., gaining weight by future and present fathers. In my case, caring for my son for the first three months absorbed me to such an extent that my body probably went crazy because I did everything contrary to the rules I had previously adopted. However, I did not feel bad about it. My son came first at that time. And he is the first today, of course. But you probably know what I mean. You might ask what took so much time? First of all, feeding and struggling to support lactation. From the very beginning, we knew that the best thing for the baby would be breastfeeding.

For this reason, we were often nursing our son and tried to stimulate sucking breast for the milk supply to kick in. The second day after hospital discharge, we were visited by an environmental midwife who weighed the baby, and it turned out that it did not gain weight. What is even worse – the weight decreased compared to the last weighing in the hospital. You should know that it is normal for the baby to lose about 10-15% of its birth weight during the first 2-3 days, then the baby gains weight and reaches birth weight in 10-14 days. We urgently found a lactation consultant (it is a pity that such services are not available in the hospital) who gave us directions by phone and visited us at home after a few days. As it turned out, our little boy sucked the breast but did not eat effectively because, due to prematurity and low birth weight, he was not strong enough and could not grasp the nipple deep enough with his mouth. Besides, my wife's lactation was very weak, so we had to get it started. Many women give up at this stage, but we chose to fight. The consultant observed the baby for 2.5 hours and gave us directions. We only owe it to her that the baby eats enough food, and my wife has no problem producing it. Our typical day was as follows:

➢ feeding every 2.5-3 hours. The boy was still too young and weak to be fed at will, so we had to wake him up every time;

- ➢ weighing the boy before breastfeeding and breastfeeding for 40 minutes (20 minutes for each breast);

- ➢ weighting to see how many grams he has gained on his weight, i.e., to calculate how much he needs to be fed from the bottle (the target quantity in the first weeks is 80 ml);

- ➢ my wife started to collect food that the baby failed to suck to stimulate further lactation; first, we used a single breast pump, it took about 45 minutes (10+10, 7+7, 5+5), then it took us 20 minutes with a double breast pump;

- ➢ I prepared a bunch of feeding bottles with food collected after the previous feeding; at first, the amount of food collected was insufficient to reach 80 ml, so I made modified milk and started feeding my son.

The above cycle took about 1.5 hours for the baby to fall asleep. Then we had about an hour for ourselves, and we had to wake him up for another feeding. Breaks between feedings are measured from the start of feeding to the beginning of the next one. In the second or third week, my son had colic pains. This is the symptom of an underdeveloped digestive system. We tried to ease them with the available supplements. This is a time when a child cannot sleep because it struggles with pain, and you are unable to help. If eventually, the child falls asleep, you need to wake it up soon, as another feeding is approaching. In the second half of the second month, lactation developed sufficiently and stabilized. Thus, collecting food was no longer necessary. Unfortunately, the colic pain had not gone away yet, which is why my son was sleepless and irritable, just like his parents.

As you can see, such a chain of events makes it impossible to find time for physical activity (you lack time, and your body needs rest). Moreover, you cannot control regular, healthy meals and their preparation. In my case, this has caused some stagnation when it comes to good shape and fitness resolutions, but not regression. I think that situations like mine described above, maybe one of the many different reasons for young fathers to gain weight.

Thanks for reading! If you enjoyed this book or found it useful I'd be very grateful if you'd post a short review on Amazon. Your support really does make a difference and I read all the reviews personally so I can get your feedback and make this book even better.

Thanks again for your support!

ABOUT THE AUTHOR

Patrick A. **Simon** is the author of three amazing books and has been exploring the world of writing since 2017. Born in the early '80s, Simon embraced pedagogy as a major field of study though he still devotes his time to other areas of study, especially economics. Being a dad and having a master's degree in pedagogy, he has acquired extensive experiences throughout his life, which serves as inspiration for his books. This has also helped him to effectively communicate and connect with his readers by writing in a light and straightforward tone that people can easily read and understand.

He loves writing about topics related to paternity, budgeting and personal management. His first book *"Soon To Be DAD: Handbook For Expectant Fathers"* explores pregnancy from a male perspective. He wrote the book mainly for expectant dads who appear to be ignored during their significant other's pregnancy to help them understand the kind of experiences they will be having.

The book provides an account of his experience with his wife's pregnancy and provides tips and advice to help readers who may be going through a similar situation. As a continuation of the first book, he published his second informative book, *"Couvade Syndrome: What Male Sympathetic Pregnancy is & how you can Fight it."* While the first one focused mainly on what soon-to-be dads should expect when their partner gets pregnant, the second one took it a step further. It focused on why soon-to-be fathers are having the strange pregnancy symptoms they may be sharing with their pregnant partners.

Another field of interest that Simon explores through his writing is family budgeting and personal money management. Based on his experiences in life as an involved father and husband, as well as his profound understanding of economics, especially budgeting, he has also devoted significant attention to household budgeting. His short e-book *"Family budgeting: Guide to Managing Household Finance"* was written to help families make the best use of the money they have, and ensure proper management of their finances without major hiccups due to overspending.

Currently, Simon is working on his fourth book on personal finance which will provide excellent tips for individuals with low income to help them manage their finances effectively. Although he is not a professional in this field, his extensive experience with money management, both in times of crisis and abundance, has prepared him for many money-related disasters. He hopes to help his readers to be prepared as well.

These delightful books are fun to read and come right from the heart of someone who has experienced all of these things first-hand. They are his perspective on various aspects of family and parenthood, which would help his readers understand their familial commitments better and be in the best position to fulfill their responsibilities. Undoubtedly, the books are a true family necessity!

Apart from writing, Simon is a father who passionately devotes his free time to his son, cooking, engaging in physical activities (he loves running and plays volleyball in an amateur league), and acquiring more knowledge in the field of economy and child psychology.

Printed in Great Britain
by Amazon

24702154R00056